Did I Survive All That To Go Through This?

Connie Owens

Thank you for reading my book!

TABLE OF CONTENTS

DEDICATION

This book is dedicated to all women diagnosed with breast cancer. Some have survived it, some have not, but each and every one of you will always and forever belong to the sisterhood of breast cancer warriors!

YOU HAVE CANCER!

There are 3 words you never want to hear,
That cause instant panic and horrible fear,
You are shocked and scared and need some answers,
When the doctor reveals …… "You have CANCER!"

"Why me, Lord?" you ask out loud,
It's one in three in every crowd,
It becomes your focus night and day,
24/7 it won't go away.

You tell your friends and family,
Most are aghast in disbelief,
Whatever we can do, just let us know,
But most aren't there for the highs and lows.

The ones whom you thought would show huge support,
Surprise you now as they disappoint,
You soon face the fact that it's _your_ fight to own,
And pray for the day that this nightmare is gone.

You do what you must and endure all the pain,
Hoping in time to be healthy again,
Doctor appointments and medical bills,
Build a mountain of debt, I'm just hoping it heals!

With fingers crossed and hourly prayers,
And continued support from all those who care,
You wait for the day that this nightmare will end,
And pray never to hear those 3 words again.

Written by: Connie Owens 01/08/2023 ©

CHAPTER 1: YOU HAVE CANCER!

YOU HAVE CANCER! Yes, those 3 words can stop a clock, stop the world from turning, stop your heart! You never really think about how it would feel for a doctor to say that you have cancer. Not really. When it does happen, it's almost like being in a dream, in a fog, or watching a bad movie. This can't be real, can it? Can it????

My sister, Marsha, found out in the spring of 2022 that she needed quadruple bypass surgery. None of us knew or had any idea her health was that bad, including her! It was quite a shock and an eye opener. She asked me to please get a physical to make sure I wasn't experiencing the same thing.

I made an appointment with my primary care doctor and went for my yearly physical. I was scheduled for a mammogram since I hadn't had one in years. It's something every woman dreads like hell. Getting your boobs smashed like a pancake is not fun! In retrospect, I am so glad I did. I had neglected getting mammograms for years. I wish now that I had gone annually. This problem could have been detected earlier, and maybe I wouldn't be dealing with all this treatment now. You just can't fix stupid.

Two days later I received a call to come back in for a follow-up mammogram because something was concerning in my right breast. Oh hell! Immediately my body froze in fear because I suspected where this could be going.

The appointment was scheduled for another mammogram of right breast only and an ultrasound. The results were what I expected and dreaded. They said, "There's something there that needs further investigation." Sure, there is!

What else did I expect to hear this day?

The mammograms and ultrasound were sent to the breast imaging office, and I was scheduled for a biopsy. <u>BIOPSY!</u> Dear Lord! This is getting very serious. If I'm in a nightmare, I sure wish that I would wake up. Hey, this isn't funny anymore!

The mere thought of someone slicing and dicing my boob was a little unnerving, but I was willing to do it so we could confirm whether it was a cyst, tumor, or exactly what. The moment of truth was here.

I was quite nervous. Thank goodness my sister, Marsha, came with me today. The staff made me feel very comfortable and at ease. Perhaps this wouldn't be as bad as I had feared it would be. A mammogram had to be done first, and then I was given an injection of something to numb the area. I felt nothing; absolutely nothing. Thank God! Of course, in my mind I was waiting for some terrible pain to start happening. I'm such a sissy.

The doctor took several samples to send to the lab. He then inserted 2 titanium markers, one in my breast, and the other in my lymph nodes. These would show up on future mammograms to mark where breast tissue had been investigated in the past. Another mammogram was taken to show where the markers were located.

The biopsy procedures were complete, and now we wait for the pathology report. I asked the doctor if he could tell if it was a cyst, and he said it definitely was <u>not</u> a cyst. He would have the results in a few days. That was frightening to hear. If there was ever a time that one would need a stiff shot of liquor, it would be now! Hmm!

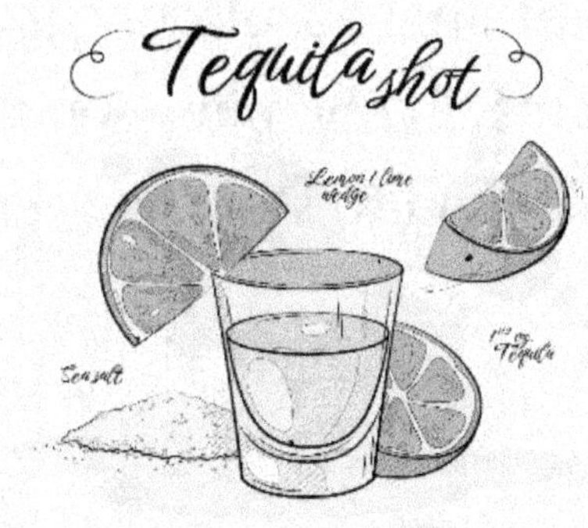

Ok, so if it's definitely not a cyst, are there other options? This can only mean one thing, right? Would I be doing all these tests if they didn't suspect "you know what??"

The next day I got a call to discuss the results. **_Carcinoma, cancer, tumor_**. All those words you just hope to never hear were coming out of my doctor's mouth. **_Second stage invasive ductal carcinoma metastatic to lymph nodes!_**

WHAT? That sounds like a death sentence; like dooms day is upon me; like the end. INVASIVE? It scared and upset me, but I held on and didn't completely lose my mind. Suddenly it was as if I were drifting away in space, and the doctor's voice kept getting farther away. I was completely swept away in the moment, but I snapped back and listened to what he was saying. He said an oncologist would further explain and let me know how we proceed from here.

I hung up the phone and just sat there alone for 30 minutes trying to soak all this in. I was in total shock, numb to the bone. How can this be? No one ever wants to get that phone call.

I had the shock of my life. The question lingered in my mind constantly, 'Where do we go from here?' I knew about breast cancer treatments, but I had no idea really what it entailed. There must be a way for me to beat this. There just must be. Right?

An appointment was made for me to see a medical oncologist in 2 days. So as this unfolds, I continued to "wait and see." With the weight of the world on my shoulders I did just that, waited for two days to see what I had to do next. I debated if I wanted to do all these treatments, yet I knew full well that there was no other option but to do it. Let's be realistic. With reluctant confidence I convinced myself that I am a strong woman, and I can do this! Can't I?

Now I had to tell my daughter, my family, and my closest friends. How would they react? I didn't want anyone to cry about it because I hadn't. Certainly some concern and empathy would be appreciated, but pity and drama were the last things I needed in an already clouded state of emotion. I already knew a lot of prayers, fingers crossed, and moral support would be tremendously encouraging. With friends and family in my corner, I can and will fight this! I'm a **_survivor,_** and I knew this would not defeat me!

How did I know that? Before we get into all the cancer drama, let's go back. I'll explain what else I survived a few years ago.

On April 16, 2011, a series of tornados swept across North Carolina. I was unknowingly in the path of an EF3 tornado that came through Snow Hill, NC. I was at home minding my own business when all hell broke loose. As I have said many times, "Riding inside a tornado was never on my bucket list!" Nope, not at all something I had yearned to do. On that particular day, I did that very thing. It picked up my house several times and tossed it like a rag doll with me inside. The sounds and smells will stick with me forever. It was the single most frightening day of my life. That few minutes suspended in time changed my life forever. It's amazing how a split second can alter a life.

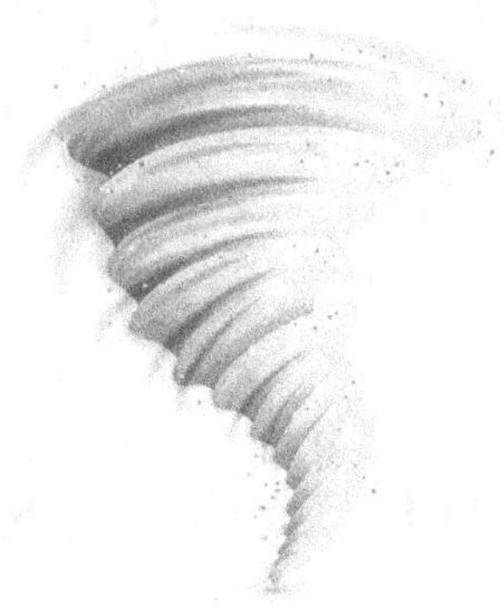

In the immediate aftermath, I was in shock. As time went on, I was a nervous wreck, depressed, jacked up, and could not relax or sleep. My emotions were all over the place. I just wanted to hide from everyone and everything. It was recommended that I see a therapist to try to understand what was going on with me. I didn't have great expectations about it at first, but soon after I was diagnosed with PTSD. Really? Me? Oh, too be sure...not me! Unfortunately, it was true. My life was totally changed, and I had to learn to cope with it.

I really tried to continue working, but I was a nervous wreck all the time. It was evident that I could no longer cope or function in a working environment. I had no choice but to go on full disability because my nerves were so bad. Sudden loud noises set me into panic mode. Bad weather and threat of storms sent me into a tailspin. I didn't want to go out with friends anymore. When invited out I would come up with a reason that I couldn't go because I just couldn't do it. I just wanted to stay home where it was safe and most of all QUIET. I was always very much a people person and enjoyed socializing and meeting new people. I was never timid or bashful by any means, and everyone remembers me! Ha! PTSD altered my very existence in many ways. I basically became a "hermit."

After turning down many invitations, soon there were none. People eventually stopped calling and asking me to do anything. I hated that, but I just couldn't help it. I became lonelier than ever and was forced to live with that choice. The solitude, serenity, and sense of safety I felt held me captive in my own home.

You have never known fear until you witness first-hand the unfathomable power of a tornado. You have ZERO control of the situation, and there is absolutely nothing you can do but pray! Being pushed beyond your limits by that kind of power creates pure, unharnessed fear that surpasses verbal description. After an experience of this magnitude, nothing can frighten you. NOTHING!

After several visits with my therapist, I told her I was beginning to remember things that I had forgotten. She said to write them down as I remembered them. I told her it was becoming a long list, enough to fill a book. She said, "Then write a book about it." Hmmm, me write a book?

I had never written a book or even thought about it. My therapist planted the seed, so I investigated how to go about starting a book. In a few short months, I had written and released a book entitled *On The Inside Looking Out*. The book was published and became available on Amazon, Books a Million, Barnes & Noble, and other online stores. It was a great stress reliever for me to document my experience and good information for others trying to cope with PTSD.

Putting pen to paper made the feelings I was experiencing come flooding out of my system. It felt good, it made me feel better, and it was the best therapy for me.

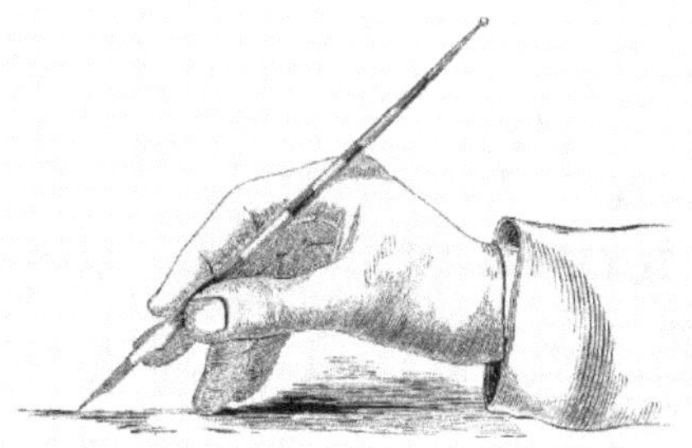

Many people including doctors and therapists have said the book gave them a broader understanding of the effects that PTSD unleashes on a family member or a patient. It helped them better understand their actions and reactions to certain situations. It offered some explanation as to why they just wanted to be left alone and not participate in anything that involved a crowd of people.

For those of you who are familiar with my first book, you can understand how the news about cancer was so devastating to me. For those not familiar, please get a copy. You will see how going *through all that (the tornado) and surviving, is helping me to survive all this (breast cancer).*

How did I survive a tornado when it could have easily taken my life that day? Was I spared to only find out 12 years later that I have breast cancer? Maybe I am just one very lucky woman. I hope and pray I can be that lucky this time.

That horrifying experience made me much stronger and more resilient. As a result, my ability to cope with just about anything thrown my way has flourished. SO, BRING IT ON! I'm a survivor, I'm invincible, and I'm capable of handling any situation. If that tornado didn't get me, do you think cancer will? I don't think so. I'll fight it until my last breath! I get up every morning ready to kick some cancer butt. It doesn't care how bad I feel!

The tornado could have taken my life, yet it only took material possessions from me. I lost 2 vehicles, my home, and everything in it. The cancer may take my life, but my material possessions will be left behind. Hmmm. Deep.

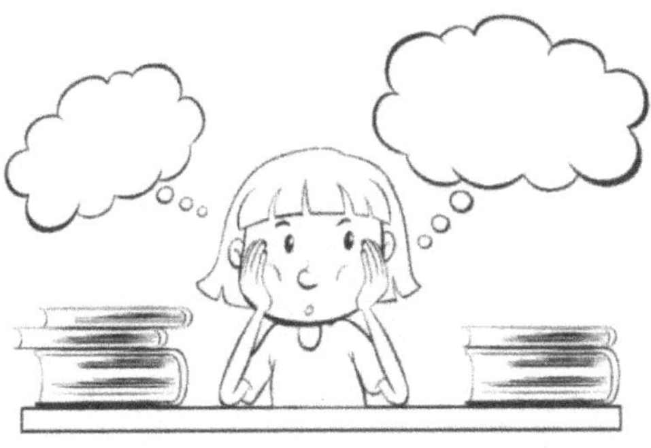

What's Next You Ask

What's next you ask, in a life full of trauma,
Do you think I need or want all the drama?
I just want peace, that's all I ask,
Is it possible? Will it come to pass?

What's next you ask, when you hear the news,
I can take it. I'm not going to lose,
Chemo and drugs then radiation,
Let's get started, no deviation.

What's next you ask, when they draw your blood,
Good results or will it be a dud?
A glimmer of hope I need today,
I want this thing to go away!

What's next you ask when surgery is done,
Did you get it all, is that battle won?
Time will tell, nothing is fast,
I can wait……. what's next you ask.

Written by: Connie Owens   June 23, 2023 ©

CHAPTER 2: WHAT'S NEXT?

The time had come to meet with the oncologist. My sister, Cheryl, came and spent the night and went with me for my first visit. When I arrived at the oncology department, they did blood work and then asked me to wait to see the doctor. As I waited, I observed other women in the waiting room. Some looked pale, some had lost all their hair, and some needed someone to support them as they walked. I sat there becoming more anxious as I envisioned myself looking like this in the months to come. Poor me. Will I look like that soon?

The doctor was very frank and to the point as she reviewed the biopsy report with me. I asked if I could survive this, and she replied, "most definitely." The treatment plan began almost immediately. I was engaged and ready to complete the recommended requirements to ensure that I survived this cancer.

The doctor opted to prescribe chemotherapy pills instead of intravenous chemo. She thought the regimen of pills would be the better therapy for me.

An appointment was scheduled to do a bone scan to see if cancer was hiding anywhere else in my body. That was frightening to hear. Could it be spread all over? Was I a goner?

My daughter, Rebecca, went with me for moral support, thank goodness. When I arrived they put an IV port in my arm and injected a dose of radioactive dye into it. I had to wait 2 hours so the dye could travel throughout my body before they could begin the scan. I wondered if I would light up like a neon sign, but it didn't happen. Would I feel like I was on fire or start to burn? I didn't feel anything any different.

While I was waiting for those 2 hours to pass, they called me in for a CT scan of my chest and abdomen. Preceding this scan, I had to drink 2 cups of something that tasted like Gatorade and yuck. As others in the waiting room sipped slowly on their cups, I chugged those 2 cups like a pro! Not a problem. (I did not crush the cups!) Ha!

An injection of contrast was next on the agenda, and the same port that was placed in my arm earlier was used. They asked if I had ever had an allergic reaction to contrast. I told them I had never had it before so I didn't know. I had to sign a form to give consent. My God, do I really have to do all this? This is going to be quite stressful, but I must do it, I just must.

As I handed the consent form back to the nurse, I wondered how many people have signed this form, received the injection, and then found out afterwards they were allergic to contrast.

The CT scan was quick. No allergic reaction or abnormalities occurred. I admit I was anticipating something weird to happen after the injection of contrast. The girl in *The Exorcist* came to mind with all her twisting, writhing, and buckling. I never felt anything. I dressed and went back to the waiting room.

After an hour delay, I was called back for the bone scan. I had to lie on a hard table for 45 minutes while the machine scanned my entire body searching for signs of cancer. It wasn't fun, but it didn't hurt. A million things go through your mind while this is happening. I was so afraid they would find more cancer somewhere else.

All the test were completed, and I impatiently waited for results. The next day I was informed that the tests revealed NO other cancer was detected. Whew! That was great to hear!

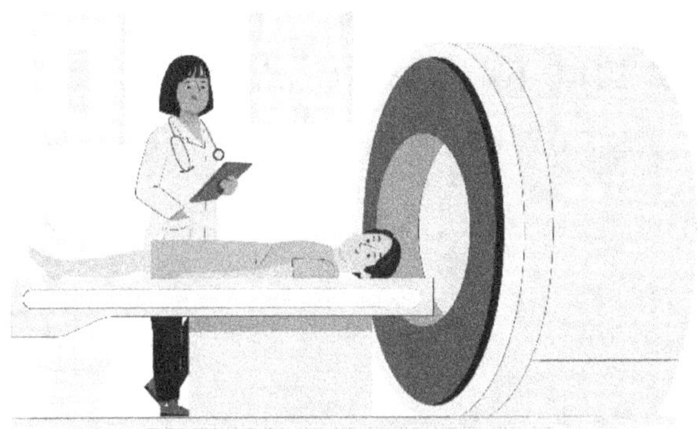

My oncologist decided to put me on Ibrance and Letrozole for 6 months. Ibrance is a targeted therapy drug known as a CDK 4/6 inhibitor. It is not a traditional chemotherapy, but when combined with certain hormonal therapies, it helps slow growth in both healthy cells and cancer cells. Although Ibrance helps to slow the progression of cancer, it has some serious side effects. I began to notice some in the 2nd month.

My side effects included: tiredness and extreme fatigue, generally feeling weak, nausea, hair thinning, shortness of breath, and coughing. I never got sick, but I was overcome with nausea several times. My biggest complaint was the fatigue and the sluggishness. My instructions were to take Ibrance for 3 weeks and then take a week off. By the middle of the second week, I became so weak I could hardly walk from room to room.

I couldn't even load or unload the dishwasher, never mind the dust mop, vacuum, or lawn mower. Just leaving my house was an ordeal. It became increasingly more apparent that everything would simply have to wait until I got my strength back. I hated this feeling, but if this is the worst it gets, then I can handle it. At least I hope so.

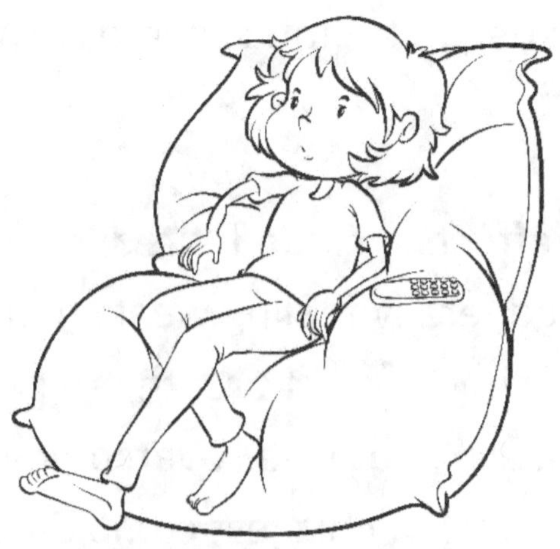

The fatigue resulted from Ibrance causing low white and red blood cell counts. By taking the 4th week off, it allowed your body to rebuild your blood counts back up to an acceptable range. Then you start all over again.

Letrozole is a nonsteroidal aromatase inhibitor. It decreases the amount of estrogen that the body produces. It can slow or stop the progression of some types of breast cancer cells, especially the ones that need estrogen to grow. Letrozole comes with its own set of side effects and, of course, I had some of those as well.

Among those were blurry vision, headaches, night sweats, and difficulty sleeping. My blurred vision became double vision at times which concerned my oncologist. She scheduled a brain CT scan immediately. That caused more worry for me thinking it had spread to my brain. My poor brain!

I found myself once again, nervous as hell, going into the CT scan room. I joked with them that the scan would be blank since there was not much brain up there, but I knew it was no laughing matter. I prayed to God that it would be a clean scan.

A phone call the next day verified that the scan was good. There were no signs of anything to be alarmed about. Thank you, thank you, thank you!

I continued seeing my oncologist once a month, during the next 6 months for lab work and follow ups. Early on, she set up an appointment for me to see a breast cancer surgeon. Surgery would be the next phase after I finished chemo drugs.

My visit to the surgeon's office was a great experience. Everyone was so professional and courteous. There was no long wait in the waiting room, less than 10 minutes. He examined me and agreed with the oncologist for 6 months of the pills prescribed. After that I was to come back to see him to set up the surgery date.

I must say that all the offices that I have visited during this ordeal have been outstanding so far. These include my primary care doctor, my oncologist, and breast imaging offices. The diagnosis and screening services performed X-rays, CT scans, ultrasounds, bone scan, and bone density test. The in-house lab and pharmacy were pleasant and prompt as well.

All are timely, professional, courteous, and make me feel comfortable. Wait time is less than 15 minutes in all these departments. I especially enjoy that they are punctual.

I Did It!

I did it, and don't I feel good?
I finished this round and I was hoping I could,
For over 6 months it was 2 pills a day,
Hoping to keep this cancer at bay.

There were days I felt really bad,
But never got sick and for that I'm glad,
I've lost some hair, it's very thin,
But I know it'll grow back again.

I didn't lose weight, and wish that I had,
I was always tired and that made me so sad,
Did all they asked through the ups and downs,
Now onward we go for the second round.

Written by Connie Owens: June 2023 ©

CHAPTER 3: I DID IT!

I did it! I got through Round 1 of this journey which included all the scans, mammograms, blood work, X-rays, biopsy, lab results, doctor visits, diagnosis, and treatment.

I started taking Ibrance and Letrozole in November of 2022. In February of 2023, neither my oncologist nor I could feel the tumors! How exciting was that? She ordered another mammogram to see if the meds I had been taking had made a difference.

Not looking forward to another crushing of the boob, but I was most anxious to see the results. Please! Please! Please let it show a significant change! It was obvious that it had shrunk just by feeling for it.

The next day I got the report and the images that revealed it had decreased in size by 50%! Yay!! I'll take 50%. YEAH! All the daily prayers and encouragement that I had received from friends, family, and even strangers were working for sure. Keep them coming!

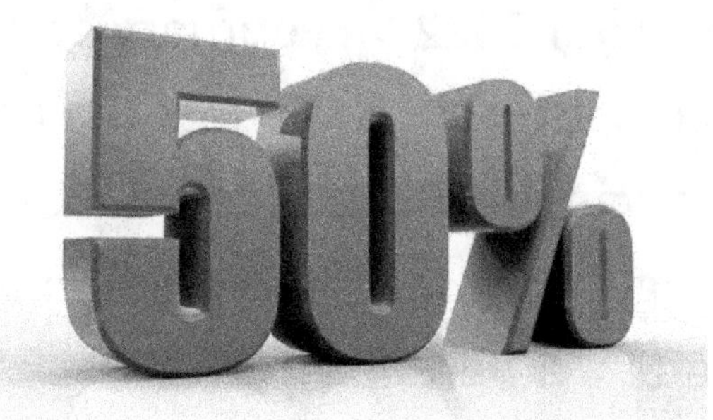

My oncologist was as excited as I was, and she instructed me to continue taking my meds for another 3 months. Geez, I hated to hear that. Although it makes me feel bad, at least I know it's working so I don't mind continuing with it. If the results in 3 more months are this good, then it will all be worth it.

It is now May of 2023. After 6 months of feeling tired and like crap regularly, and my hair thinning and falling out daily, I finally finished taking Ibrance and Letrozole. Praise the Lord! My hair was thinning so much it began to worry me. My sister, Cheryl, ordered a wig that looks very much like my hair just in case it might be needed.

The time has come to see the breast surgeon to schedule my surgery. Gulp! Here I go with the nerves again. Anxiety is high about going under the knife, but I'm still very excited to get this OUT OF MY BODY. Get this invasive thing out before it attacks my entire body. I want it gone; you hear me?? GONE!

My surgery was scheduled for May 26. This wait-and-see game brought on pacing, nervousness, fidgeting, can't sleep or rest, and envisioning all sorts of things that may or may not happen. Anyone facing surgery has similar random thoughts. Even when you're not thinking about it, you realize your brain still is.

My best friend, Jackie, came and stayed with me to drive me to surgery and take care of me afterwards. On the morning of the surgery, I had to go back to the breast imaging office first. It was the same location where the biopsy was done. The procedure today was to have a wire inserted that indicated where the biopsy was done. A wire! A damn wire! Inserted into the breast?? Lord, please get me through this day!

It was the same doctor who did my biopsy. Once again I felt nothing after he numbed the area. I saw it all happen on a monitor. The doctor said to just let him know if I felt anything, and he would numb it more. I told him not to worry, I would definitely let him know!

I lay there all pinched up and tense waiting for excruciating pain while watching the monitor and seeing that wire being inserted. I felt a little faint and light headed seeing all that, but it was over quickly, and I really didn't feel anything.

Another mammogram confirmed for the surgeon that the wire was properly inserted. It looked weird to see that wire in there. The human body can certainly take a lot of abuse.

Those very necessary pre-op requirements didn't take long so we went over to sign in for my surgery. Someone please cue the music from *Jaws!* You know that eerie bass tune that played every time the shark was lurking nearby in the shadows. That is exactly how I felt inside. I was scared, but I knew this had to happen. I bet you are hearing that music now, aren't you? As I wrote this I heard it also, and it stuck in my head for the remainder of the day. Geez. Sorry.

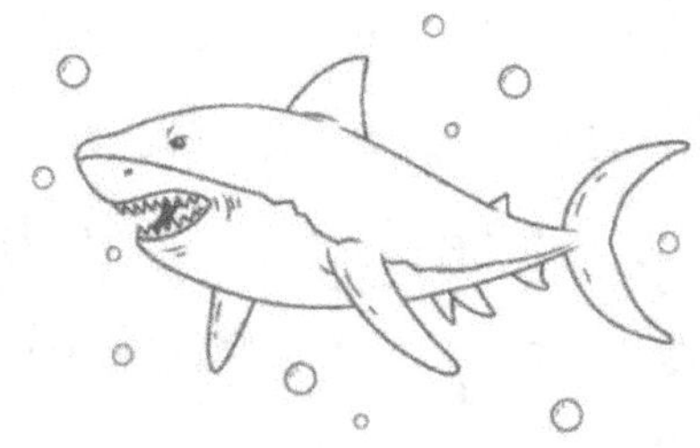

I signed in, got my hospital bracelet, and waited to be called back. My sister, Marsha, had just arrived to wait with Jackie when I was called back for "prep." Gulp, prep??? What in the world will this entail?

A lot of questions were asked. The questionnaire involved medical and family history, current prescriptions, and so on. Then I was given a gown, compression leggings, and the infamous cap. How festive I looked. Not!

An IV port was inserted into the top of my left hand. Ouch, that didn't feel good at all. Probably the worst pain I have felt to date. The anesthesiologist came in to review what he would do and to ask me some other questions.

Surgery time was approaching quickly. My anxiety had calmed down somewhat until I heard what was about to happen next.

The nurse informed me that the doctor would come in before I went into surgery and inject some blue radioactive dye into......wait for it.... are you ready? M**y nipple**! Huh? What did she just say? **Oh Lord have mercy on my soul!** Heaven forbid! Surely, she did not just say that! No Way! Is it too late to escape this joint? Waaa!!

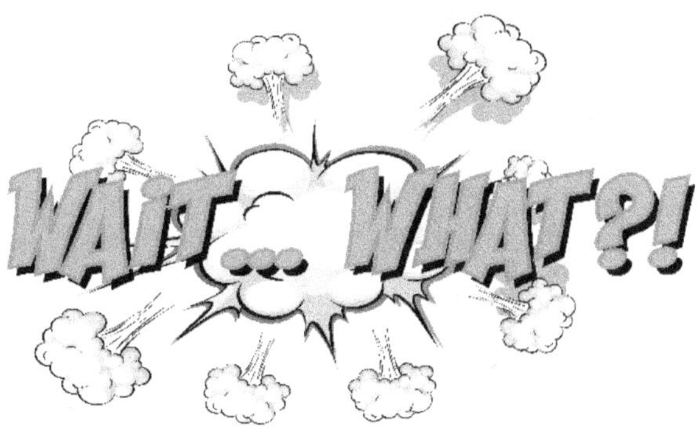

It hurt me just hearing her tell what he was preparing to do, but she added that I would get a shot of "joy juice" in my port before he came in to help relax me. Relax me? Who in the hell could be relaxed with this about to happen? Uh, yeah, please relax me. I felt a major panic attack was about to seize upon me. Somehow, I maintained.

Marsha and Jackie joined me in prep, and I told them what was going to happen. I could see they both felt the same "oh, hell no" as me. The look on their faces said it all.

The nurse injected the "joy juice", and it didn't take long at all for it to kick in. I got the silly giggles, and everyone was laughing. That was some good stuff! And boy, did I need it!

When the doctor came in, all visitors were asked to step out because of the radioactive dye. I don't think anyone had to ask either of them twice to leave before this procedure. No one would want to witness that! Thank goodness I had that shot because I just didn't even care at that moment.

The next thing I remembered was asking Marsha and Jackie, "When is he going to do it?" They both laughed and said that he had already done it. I remember the doctor coming in, but I don't remember the injection. Not at all. Thank you, Jesus, for that!

The purpose of the blue radioactive dye was to drain from the original tumor into the axillary lymph nodes in my arm pit that had cancer cells. The surgeon would then know which axillary lymph nodes needed to be removed. The end result was the removal of 17 to be sure he had gotten all the cancer cells. I didn't even know there were so many under your arm, but I found out it is usually between 20 and 49.

Ok, here comes the surgery room crew. Once again cue the music from *Jaws*. I heard that sinister tuba rumbling loud and clear as I traveled briskly down the hall, counting the overhead lights, and coming to an abrupt halt in the operating room.

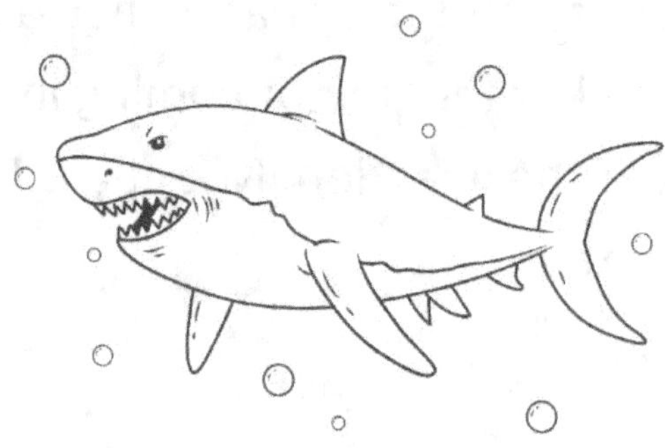

The operating room staff was very friendly and made me feel at ease. They even put a warm blanket on me. It was as cold as a meat locker in there. A blood pressure cuff was put on my left arm, and I was told they would use the same IV port that I had inserted earlier. They said that I'd be asleep soon. As they scurried around making final preparations, I lay there looking at the ceiling wondering how long it would take. It didn't take long. So now this is it, another moment of truth. I hope in a few hours when I wake up in recovery, I'll find out that the surgeon got it all.

The next thing I knew, I heard someone saying, "Hello, Ms. Owens. How are you feeling?" Huh? Where am I? Feeling? Feeling what? Then it dawned on me that it was over, and I was in the recovery room. I had some pain under my arm and the nurse gave me something to help alleviate that.

I heard more voices. Marsha and Jackie were saying, "You did it! You came through it just fine." They said the doctor told them he was sure he got it all.

I was thinking, this wasn't as bad as I had imagined it would be. Whew, I'm glad that part is over! I knew it wouldn't be long before I could go home. It was time for recovery.

In a short while the nurse said I could get dressed. As quick as Superman could don his cape, I was dressed and signing release forms. A wheel chair was brought over, Jackie left to get the car, and I was whisked down the hall to the exit door! Bye, it's been fun. See ya!

Wow? Is this really over this quickly? In a flash I was in the car and heading home. Whoa! Please stop and get me something to eat. I haven't eaten since 7:00 last night! God bless Chick-fil-A!

It's Time To Recover

Check in and prep, I'm watching that clock,
It's surgery at ten, oh my tick tock,
The doctor steps in, to encourage the day,
The surgical team comes to whisk me away.

It sure is cold in this big bright room,
It's all ok, it'll be over soon,
They put me at ease, then put me to sleep,
I pray the Lord my soul to keep.

The next thing I know, I open my eyes,
I'm now in recovery and they want me to rise,
I'm feeling some pain, but it's not for long,
Get up and get dressed, prepare to go home.

It's time to recover, the surgery is done,
It wasn't that bad, but it sure wasn't fun,
I dreaded this day, although it went fast,
It's time to recover and heal at last.

WRITTEN BY CONNIE OWENS: JUNE 2023 ©

CHAPTER 4: TIME TO RECOVER

Round 1 was diagnosis and chemotherapy. Round 2 was surgery. Now Round 3 is recovery and preparing for Round 4 which will be radiation.

So far, although none of this has been a picnic, it has been quite tolerable. I'm dreading the radiation since I must go for 7 weeks, 5 days a week. Ugh. But first I've got to heal from this surgery.

I finally arrived at home after surgery, and I was still a little sleepy. I was also wired up from all the morning activity so I didn't sleep until that night. I slept in my recliner for days because I had a drain tube in my arm pit. I was afraid I would roll over and jerk it out, smash it, clog it up, or roll over on it and hurt myself. I was less likely to move around in the recliner than in an actual bed.

The drain bulb had to be emptied and the amount drained was documented initially about every 4 hours. The tube going into my arm pit was more painful than the actual surgical site. Every movement felt like it was pulling out. It was very tender, especially where the drain tube was attached. Needless to say, I moved very cautiously and gently. I certainly didn't want anything like that to happen.

Jackie was so attentive helping with the drain tube, tracking my meds, and preparing meals. I didn't want to burden her, but I sure was glad she came. This was all very scary, and I didn't want to be alone. She lives 100 miles away and had to return after 4 days. I wish she lived closer for convenience if I need her for anything, but that simply isn't a long-term option.

My sister, Marsha, lives next door, and she brought over meals and checked on me. From time to time, she would bring a little gift or something special. I was okay by myself most of the time; lonely and worried, but okay. Within a few days I could empty the drain tube and document the amount for myself. I was still very weak and had no energy to do much of anything. Thank goodness I didn't have to go anywhere. I could just sit here in this recliner and let my body heal. Everything else going on in the world had to take care of itself for a while.

My yard has needed some serious attention. Grass needed mowing, weeds came up everywhere, shrubs needed cutting, needed weed eating, etc. All that would just have to wait. It was physically impossible for me to do it. I have two friends, Jackie and Brian, who volunteered to help me with various yardwork. Thank you!

Lots of friends texted and called and checked on me throughout this ordeal. They were very encouraging and supportive. Some friends have really gone above and beyond to help cheer me up and kept encouraging me that everything was going to be alright. Jackie has called me <u>every</u> single day since this began. My friend, Peggy, has been through all this before, and she has been my best source for knowing in advance what to expect. When you are in a health crisis, sometimes these kind gestures make all the difference in the world.

When you have cancer it's on your mind day and night. From the time you get up in the morning until you go to bed at night, it occupies your mind all day. Every time you notice the least little twinge that feels different, the first thought that comes to mind is, 'Damn I bet that cancer has moved somewhere else. Has it spread??'

These thoughts that continue to enter your mind will wear you completely out. The long-term daily grind of feeling sickly and weak, nausea, pain, and all the long list of side effects creates a perfect storm for the onset of anxiety and depression. Some days I wouldn't hear from anyone and often wondered if everyone had forgotten what I have recently endured, not to mention what I'm still facing.

Just a quick text, an email, a phone call, or a card through the mail makes all the difference in the world to someone who feels like the world is spinning without them.

It was a hard fight for me to keep myself from being pulled down into a black abyss of dark depression and a big job just to maintain some positivity in my current situation. I told myself that 'everyone is busy with their own lives.'

This cancer business is with me 24/7. Others

think about it when they "think" about it. It doesn't possess their mind like it does mine. I'll be glad when life returns to normal for me and I don't think about cancer, cancer, cancer all the time.

Bottom line is that I'm the sick one here. It's my fight to own, and I have accepted that. I will fight to survive this with all that I have. I will get better, and I will start living life again, real soon, I hope. Enough of the pity party. Let's move on.

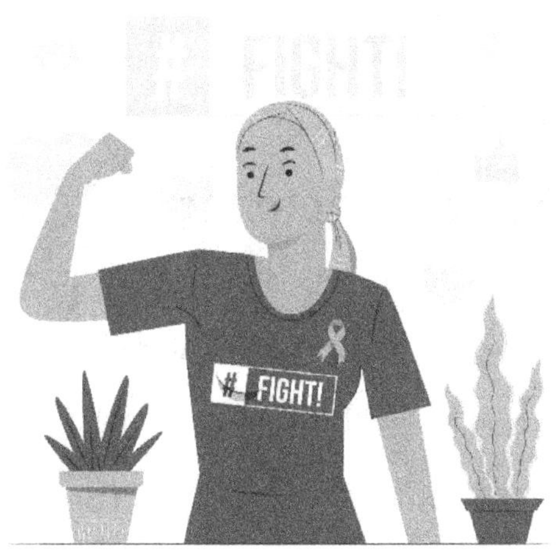

A week after surgery my sister, Cheryl, took me back to the surgeon's office for a post-op checkup. I was dreading this because of the probability that the drain tube would be removed. I wondered if it would feel like my insides were being pulled out or being gutted like a fish. Hey, I admit that I'm a big sissy. I anticipate that everything is going to hurt like hell. The nurse came in and checked my drain tube. Her assessment was that I had to keep it in another week and to continue documenting the amount. Yay, but damn! I had mixed emotions about it, but I was sure hoping to get rid of that aggravating ball and chain today.

The surgeon came into the exam room with a smile. "I'm pretty sure we got it all", he reported. He reviewed the pathology report with me and kept emphasizing "NO TUMOR FOUND." Yay! This means, according to the pathology lab, that no cancer cells were found in the areas beyond the tumors he removed.

He had discussed with me that he would remove a sizable amount of tissue around the tumors to ensure that he got all the cancer cells. The report also stated that the 17 lymph nodes he removed had no cancer. So I asked him if I was cancer free and he said yes, I was. As of this moment in time, in the general breast area, I was cancer free! He checked my incision and said it was healing beautifully and that I came through the surgery great, but I must continue to rest and not overdo until it healed and I got my strength back.

The surgeon made an appointment for me to see the radiation oncologist and arrange the schedule for radiation treatments. I asked when the appointment was, and he said, "Right now". Somewhat bewildered I responded, "Oh, I didn't know I had this appointment today. I have to meet with my medical oncologist in 3 hours, but I should have enough time." He also made an appointment to check my drain the following week.

I crossed the road to the radiation/oncology department at the hospital and checked in. The nurse took me back and asked all those same questions you are asked at every doctor's office about medical history, family history and other redundant stuff. The repetition gets tiresome but I know each office needs its own records.

The radiation oncologist came in and introduced himself to me. He examined me and checked my incision. He then discussed in some detail what radiation was, why we do it, and what my treatment would consist of. I was nervous, but he put my mind at ease. He said I would get 34 radiation treatments, five days a week for seven weeks. The first week would only be 4 days. Everyone in his office from check-in to check-out was very nice and professional. No one had any snarky attitude like you get sometime at doctor's offices. You know what I'm talking about. We've all been there and done that.

We left there with an abundance of information about radiation and an appointment for the next week to get "mapped and tattooed." Gulp! That sounds scary and not something I was looking forward to.

We had a quick drive-thru lunch before heading to the oncologist's office. By this time, I'm extremely exhausted. I didn't realize all this was planned. The radiologist appointment was something I had to deal with today unexpectedly, but we're here so why not?

My oncologist came into the room smiling and excited to read the pathology report. She agreed that the incision looked great and was healing nicely. She now wanted to discuss what would happen after I finished my radiation treatments.

The oncologist said she was on the fence about

giving me a couple of rounds of intravenous chemo, but considering my age (eye roll), sticking with the pills would be the best option. After I finish with my radiation treatments, she will prescribe Letrozole and Verzenio, as a precaution. Since Letrozole, the estrogen blocker, did its job previously, she thought it would be wise to stay on that for a while. Instead of taking Ibrance, like I did before surgery, I would be taking Verzenio. I'll find out more about taking these meds at my next appointment with her.

I was not looking forward to taking any more medication that would cause that sluggish, tired, run-down feeling that I had already experienced for the last six months, but if that is what is required, I'll suck it up and do it.

I arrived back home with the drain tube still intact with instructions to monitor it for yet another week. The discharge doesn't seem to be slowing down at all yet. Where the hell is all this coming from? Maybe I'll shrink a few sizes losing all this fluid. Or not! It would be great if they could invent a tube to drain the fat out of your belly! I'd sign up for that in a heartbeat! I think everyone would.

As days crawl by, I'm slowly getting my strength back little by little. I'm ready for my next doctor visit to hopefully get this tube removed. In retrospect, it's amazing how the human body can heal; that it can undergo all that trauma and bounce back as if nothing ever happened. It has become very uncomfortable dealing with this drain tube and drain bulb. I couldn't stand for my arm to touch them. I went online and searched for an arm sling or something to elevate my arm and possibly keep my arm from touching the surgical site. I found an arm sling that had a pillow attached to it that would do that very thing. I ordered one immediately and used it for several days. It helped a lot.

A week had passed, and I was on my way to see if the drain can be removed. I took my documentation sheet for them to see how much was draining. The nurse cleaned the drain tube and put a new bandage over the drain exit. I was disappointed to learn that I had to keep it yet another week. Lord, help me. Will this ever end?

One more week of wearing and monitoring this thing was about to get on my nerves, but I had to wait until post-op visit number 3. We can remove the tube today. Hip hip hooray! Wait, oh no! This is going to make me faint, I just know it is! I asked the nurse, "Has anyone ever fainted, fell off the table, hit their head, knocked themselves unconscious, and needed stitches etc. during this procedure?" She laughed and said, "Not yet." I said, "Well today could be that monumental day." It could be a day she would talk about for the rest of her career. She assured me it wasn't that bad. I was thinking, 'Yeah right, famous last words.' I was beyond ready to have this removed.

At this point I really didn't care how it felt. Well, not really. I'm lying about that. I was preparing to scream like a little school girl and probably clear the waiting room! Ha!

She told me to take a deep breath and exhale when she said the word. Voilà, it was out, gone, and I didn't faint! That was way too easy, and I got all bunched up over it for nothing. Piece of cake! Yeah, I'm tough alright. I knew that wouldn't hurt. You know that is a lie. Ha!

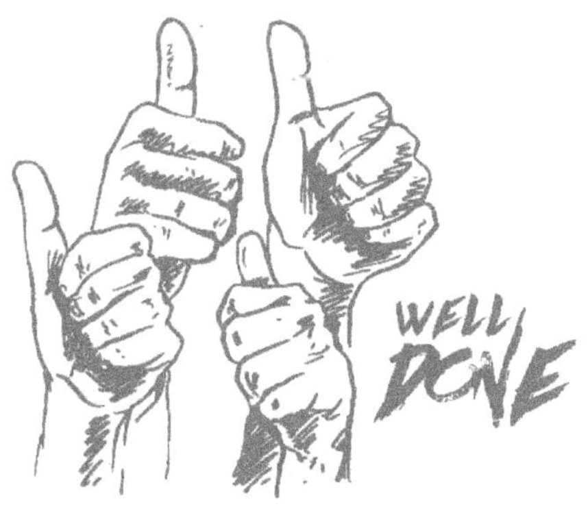

Whew, that is over, and I'm going home drain tube free. I feel so much better just knowing I don't have to deal with all that anymore. I'm ready to get back to feeling like me once more and start enjoying life again. I have been a recluse for over 6 months, staying at home, trying not to catch a cold, or the flu, or that damn Corona virus. I just didn't need anything else dragging me down right now. Dealing with the cancer was all I could handle at the present moment.

With the drain tube out, I could dress myself without fear of ripping out the tube, and I could finally sleep on my side. Yay!! It's a little tender but feels so much better than before. No more draining and documenting the tube. I have been set free!

My strength is improving but still not up to par. I get completely deflated just making my bed. Three weeks of sleeping in the recliner weren't too bad during that time. At least I didn't have to make a bed then. My appetite is good. I'm feeling a little more like venturing out of these walls. I'm so ready to go out somewhere and eat in a restaurant and relax for a while. I need to see something other than the inside of my own home.

My aunt Becky suggested we do that very thing. We went to a Hibachi restaurant that had a big buffet. I helped myself to some of everything, I think. Mercy me, this is good! What a wonderful celebration dinner! Afterwards we walked it off in Ollie's which was right next door. I didn't particularly need anything from there, but I did need to walk that dinner off! We were stuffed.

The following week I went to radiology to get "mapped and tattooed." I really didn't know what all that meant, but I was going to find out. The radiation therapist, Ashley, happened to be the sister of one of my best friends, (Brian). It's such a small world. Just knowing who she was helped to alleviate some of the anxiety.

Before you begin radiation treatment, your radiation therapy team carefully plans your treatment in a process called radiation simulation. Treatment planning usually involves positioning your body, making marks on your skin, and taking imaging scans.

First, I was positioned on the table and I had to put my arms over my head while lying flat on my back. A pillow was placed underneath my right side. Several CT images were taken of the area that would need radiation. This would help the radiation oncologist determine exactly where my treatment will be focused.

Laser lights were aimed at my body. After all the alignments were adjusted and tweaked to her satisfaction, she put marks on my skin with a permanent marker. Then a clear round plastic adhesive circle was placed over each of those marks. These marks make sure that I'm precisely positioned and aligned each time I get radiation treatments.

It would take 8 to 10 business days for them to prepare my unique treatment plan, and I would be informed when my treatments would begin. I dressed and headed home to "wait and see" yet again. After all these months, now I'm ready to get this started and finished. I've got things I want to do, places to go, people to see. Hurry up already!

Two weeks later I got a call to set up my radiation schedule. It was planned to start the following week on Tuesday at 7:45 a.m. I asked for an early appointment so I could get it done and get back home. I didn't want it interfering with my whole day.

It will be 5 days a week for 7 weeks, but that's ok. I'm just ready to get this part of my treatment behind me too.

I have a great group of friends who have promised a big celebration for my victory of being cancer free. With all the meds, tests, chemo, surgery, recovery, and radiation behind me, I can't wait for that landmark weekend. It cannot get here fast enough, but I want to be well first. I want to enjoy every minute of it. That weekend could be dangerous. We could make the news! Ha!!

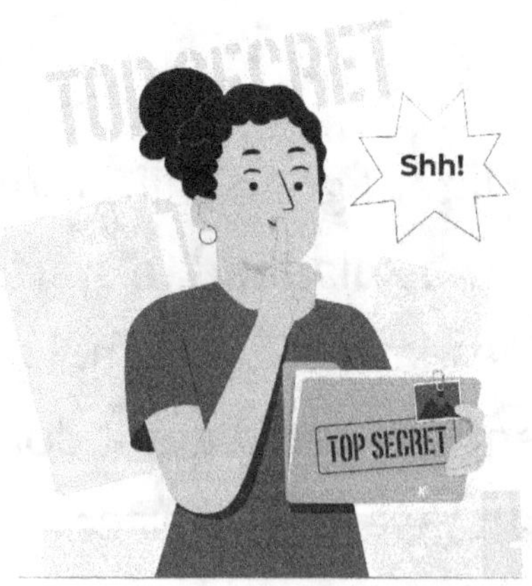

Cancer Free

Nothing about cancer is fun nor free,
Co-pays and bills, nearing bankruptcy,
A dollar here, a hundred there,
But you do anything for the proper care.

I'm a walking appointment book,
Can you come on this day, let me look,
I'm free at ten, if you can squeeze me in,
2 more this week, will it ever end?

Oncology, pharmacy, and surgery,
How much more can they do to me?
Lab work here, lab work there,
Hair falling out, need a wig to wear.

I've finished chemo, starting radiation,
I'm so tired of all this aggravation,
Cancer free! Yes, cancer free!
That's all I want them to say to me.

Written by: Connie Owens June 2023 ©

CHAPTER 5: CANCER FREE?

I am still trying to process the fact that my surgeon says I'm cancer free. Am I really? Even after hearing those words, I still have doubts. Could something still be lurking inside somewhere playing hide and seek while waiting for the big reveal? I know that sounds negative, but that's what I'm thinking. I feel sure everyone who has cancer thinks this way.

Although I am most excited and happy that the surgery is over and those tumors are gone, I still worry that the cancer might return. I wish I didn't have those thoughts, but the possibility keeps running through my brain. I hear so much about people who have cancer, finished chemo and radiation, and then they find that it has spread elsewhere. That really must be a kick in the gut.

This treatment ordeal has been quite a lengthy

process, and I'm nowhere near the end of it yet. It has been a year since I received the first mammogram indicating an area of concern. It has been an ongoing wild ride since then. I have been to the doctor more times in the past year than I have in my entire life! The appointments have not slowed down at all. If this is the schedule I must keep to be cancer free, then by all means bring it on!

The incision from surgery has healed, and it doesn't look so bad. It actually looks like a smiley face. I hope it's smiling and saying, "It's all gone! Don't worry, be happy." Damn, now that song is ringing in my head. The power of suggestion. Ugh!

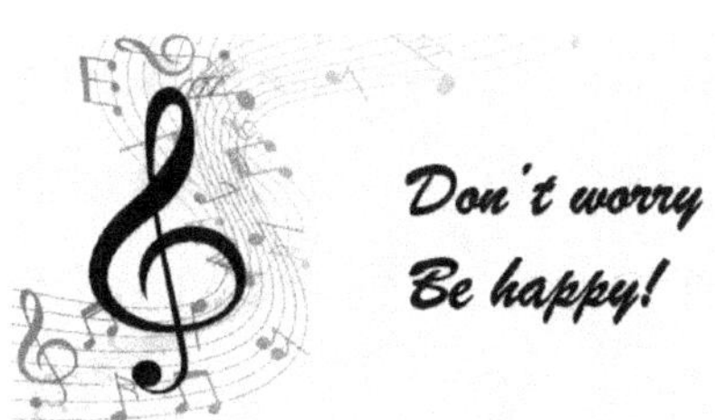

My next mammogram was scheduled in one month which is 3 months after the surgery occurred. I was a little anxious about that. You can likely imagine the thoughts going through my head as I ponder the possible results. With fingers crossed, I prayed that it would be clean and without any abnormalities.

My first radiation treatment was scheduled to begin the next morning. I wasn't really nervous at this point, but I was a little unsettled because of the unknown. Several friends who had radiation treatments have assured me that I would do okay, and it's not as bad as people think. I hope that is factual and not just words to boost my morale.

Radiation following a lumpectomy has proven to significantly reduce the risk of cancer returning in the affected breast. I feel confident that it will benefit me.

My thoughts turned to science fiction as I thought about these treatments. I envisioned laser beams aimed at a target and shattering it to smithereens. My imagination has been in overdrive, working overtime playing with my thoughts. I'll probably laugh on the way home tomorrow that I even imagined that it would be horrible. Leave it to me to overthink what the experience may be like.

As I sat here and worried myself with these crazy ideas, I decided to write more pages for this book to keep my mind occupied until bedtime. By this time tomorrow, the appointment would be done. I would know what to expect after that. It would be another new adventure into the unknown and beyond. Radiation sounds so much like entering the *Twilight Zone*. Am I there? It was going to be a long night; and I really needed sleep.

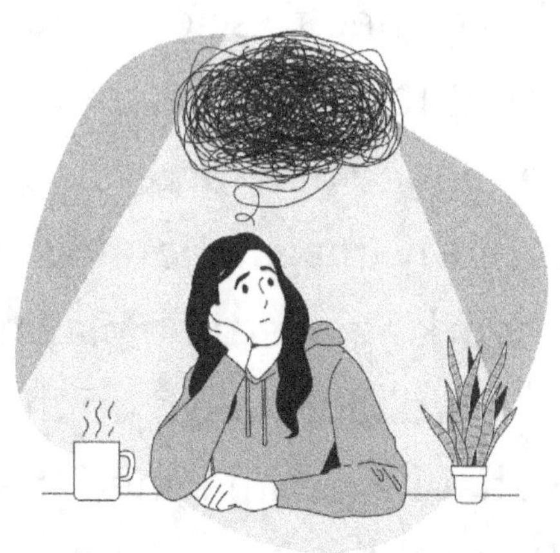

Dawn was breaking, and my first radiation treatment is today. Woohoo and yippee ki-yay! I took my sweet time getting dressed as if I was heading to the gas chamber. I'm not scared, but I am a little shaken. It's the unknown that will worry you to death. While driving to the hospital, I talked out loud rather sternly to myself. Aloud was far more emphatic. Hearing it was more encouraging than just thinking it. I was saying things like, "You can do this. Don't be a big sissy."

I arrived, checked in, and was taken to the waiting room. I was requested to put on a gown that opened in the front and someone would be out to get me shortly. In a few minutes I was called back and the radiation therapist explained everything that was going to take place. They quickly put me at ease, and in no time I was feeling better. Ashley, the sister of one of my best friends, was there. She explained more about the treatment and what to expect. I felt more comfortable just knowing someone, not just a stranger doing a job. Thank you, Ashley!

I was asked to lie on a table, and they began to position me. Those tattoos that I got several weeks ago were used to align the radiation machine precisely. My arms were up over my head as I held on to two handles while they repositioned my body until everything aligned.

They explained that the machine would circle me several times. It would not get close or touch my body. I was asked if I wanted some music playing while I was in there and I said, "Play some good ol' Carolina beach music." They made it happen! I was instructed to remain as still as possible during the treatment. I thought, not a problem! You literally couldn't have driven a mustard seed up my ass with a jack hammer at that moment! Talk about tension, whew!! I was wound up too tight! I was anticipating some bright beam of light to appear making a buzzing sound as it zapped my body, but that didn't happen.

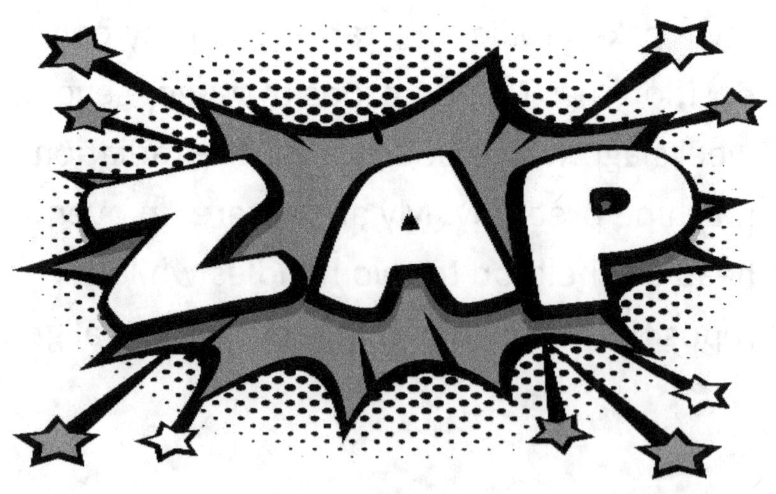

It was over before I knew what happened. I felt nothing, I saw nothing unusual; not one thing! No bright light resembling the search light over Alcatraz, no electric shock, no ray of hot laser beam frying my body. I mean NOTHING. I only heard a sound like a mosquito buzzing around my head. Other than that, nothing at all.

The therapist came in and removed the clear adhesive circles that were over my tattoo marks and made new tattoo marks. Once those were covered, I was done. They helped me off the table, but I couldn't dress yet because I would see the radiation doctor next.

The doctor wanted to know how the first treatment went and asked if I had any questions. He assured me that the treatments would go by quickly and I should do well. He suggested I may need to have some aloe vera gel on hand in a few weeks if it started to burn. We had a good discussion. He then said I could dress and leave for the day.

Easy, peasy! I had stressed myself out for nothing. Like I said, it's the unknown that will annoy you to death. Today was day one of 34 treatments, and now I know what to expect. If it all goes as smoothly as this day, this will go by quickly and I will be ok.

On the way home I was singing "Easy" by Lionel Ritchie. Driving along, making up my own words, singing, smiling ear to ear, and grateful that I had survived yet another traumatic moment during this journey. I had survived first-day jitters of radiation. Well done!

My good friend, Peggy, went through a similar treatment plan, and she has been the best support person anyone could ask for. She encouraged me last night and told me today how proud she was of me. Having someone like her in your corner absolutely helps this process move along. They know what to expect, they know what I'm going through, and they know the right things to say to support me through this journey. Thank God I have her to lean on.

Week 1 of radiation went by quickly and without issues. It has become routine, and I think overall I am going to be able to handle this just fine. I have met some new friends who are going through the same thing.

My treatment was scheduled at 7:45 every morning. Another patient whose name is Lula was always in the waiting room when I am there. After only a few short days, we talk as if we are old friends. It's amazing how that works. We were perfect strangers a week ago. Now it's like we have known each other for years. The sisterhood of survival bonds us together, and our circle has grown. We all know the deal by now, and there is no pretense or tiptoeing around each other. We just laugh and carry on. We talk about our families and how long we have been doing this. We compare "battle scars" and encourage each other to hang in there because better days are coming.

After 4 radiation treatments, I started having pain in my right shoulder when I laid down at night. My first thought was that the radiation had burned a hole through my shoulder socket! It was more severe when I got into bed and laid flat. I couldn't sleep on either side or lie on my back. The pain pounded worse than a toothache. I had to get back in the recliner to get any relief, and it took over an hour to ever go back to sleep.

Week 2 was almost over. I called my surgeon's office and described the intense shoulder pain, wondering if other patients had similar issues. The nurse said normally any complications after a lumpectomy would be tightening or pain in the chest. She suggested that I call my oncologist about the symptoms.

I called and explained the shoulder pain and discomfort from the nagging ache and the resulting inability to sleep. She said it could be coming from the positioning on the radiation table with my arms above my head. Maybe I had pulled something or just aggravated it by lying in that position. I was told to take some Advil and see if it would help with the pain.

I did that for the next 3 nights, and it still hurt me so much that I couldn't sleep in the bed. I was walking around like a zombie from lack of sleep. Something had to change. I wasn't making this stuff up. I damnit hurt!

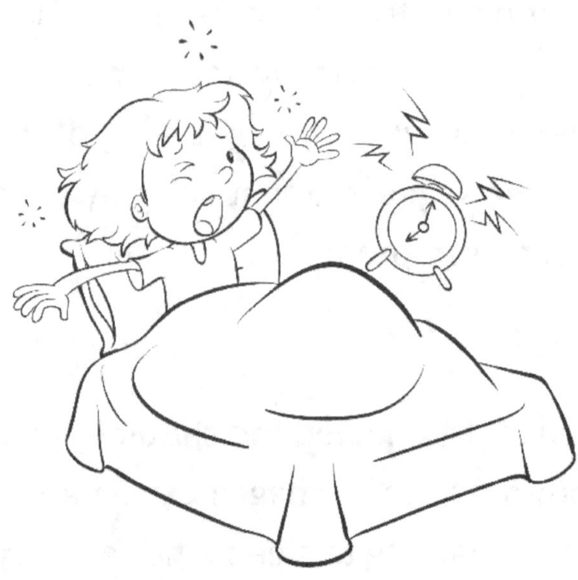

I discussed this pain with my radiation doctor. He also said it was probably from the way I had to lie on the radiation table and recommended Advil to alleviate the pain. All doctors assured me that it wasn't coming from my cancer and that it would go away on its own before I knew it. I was glad to see no one was real concerned about it. At least I felt better having discussed it with them.

The following night I took a Xanax before bed to help me fall asleep. Sure enough, I went right on to sleep. Around 1:45 I woke up with that throbbing pain again and went back to the recliner. I played this game for another 2 nights. As mysteriously as it appeared, it also disappeared. I guess I did strain something in that shoulder. I'm just glad it is gone!

I can usually handle pain very well. I generally don't complain about hurting unless I am seriously hurting. I'm sure the doctors have their share of chronic complainers who gripe about every single tiny little thing. When someone like me complains, they may just brush it off as insignificant. If I ever say that I don't feel good, I'm tired, or I hurt, you better believe I mean it.

COUNTING THE DAYS

The journey is long, and patience is short,
There are times when you just want to abort,
But you journey on and do as they say,
Keep the faith and keep counting the days.

Sooner or later, you'll get to the end,
You'll look back to where you first began,
For all you have done, you will be amazed,
You kept the faith, and kept counting the days.

Healing takes time, and cannot be rushed,
There are times when your hopes are crushed,
Take the good with the bad, remember to pray,
Hold on to faith, and keep counting the days.

When it's all over you'll look back and see,
You weren't alone, you thought you would be,
So many prayers were coming your way,
They kept the faith and kept counting the days.

Written by Connie Owens: July 2023 ©

CHAPTER 6: COUNTING THE DAYS

Week 3 I have counted each day and checked it off my calendar as this part of the journey continues. I'm almost at the halfway point of radiation treatments. It hasn't been unbearable so far. Some burning sensation began this week, but I can deal with it. As with any skin burn, after a while it begins to itch more and more. I apply hydrocortisone to soothe it. It's like a mild sunburn now, but it's in a very tender and sensitive area.

Lula had her last treatment this week, and her birthday was the next day. I bought her a little something for the occasions and put it in a festive gift bag with 2 cards. One was Congratulations on finishing radiation and the other was for her Happy 70th Birthday. She was so excited. In just this short span of time, we have become good friends. I'm going to miss seeing her every morning.

Paula, Cindy, and Fannie are in the waiting room every morning with me now. We discuss our preferred remedies to alleviate the pain, itching and discomfort. It's very helpful to hear from others who are further along in treatment. You get insight about what happens next. I can also offer helpful experience to those who are behind me in their treatment. It's such a great support team.

New women come in every week, and it doesn't take long to get into conversations and become friends. Talking to them every morning is enjoyable, and I look forward to it. I will not miss driving the 52 miles round trip every day to Greenville for radiation, but I will miss the comradery I have built with these strong women.

The receptionists at the front desk of the radiation center, Jackie and Sheena, are so nice. Both always seem to be very happy and welcome me kindly. They call me by my name saying, "Good morning, Miss Owens, I've got you checked in!" They also wish me a good day when I leave and say, "We'll see you tomorrow!" What an upbeat way to start the day!

The radiation therapists are also a joy to deal with each day. Always smiling with great attitudes, they really seem to enjoy their jobs. They greet me each morning by asking how I'm doing. They very caringly help me on and off the table, play good music during treatment, and then ask what I have planned for the rest of the day. I've had several different radiation therapists through the weeks: *Adam, Sue, Ashley, Jared, Anna, Erica, Brandi, Jennie, and Cindy.* I have enjoyed meeting each and every one of them.

I must say that the whole team here at the radiation oncology center have the greatest attitudes and treat their patients with the utmost respect. These attributes make this whole experience easier to cope with. The cheerful attitudes and professionalism displayed by all the employees make you feel more like a "friend" than a "patient" when you arrive. The weight of the world is already on your shoulders anyway because of the illness. The care and understanding shown by the staff is very comforting and helps in a big way to put patients at ease. Bravo to all of you!

Each day I hear cha-ching, cha-ching, as the bills keep piling up. Nothing about cancer treatment is cheap. There are so many steps in the process of treating it. Many visits are required to many doctors. Multiple tests are performed, including mammograms, MRIs, CT scans, bone scans, blood work, biopsy, surgery, chemotherapy, and radiation. Even with insurance my co-pay is $75 for <u>each</u> visit of 34 radiation treatments. Whew! Talk about stressing out! Where's my money tree??

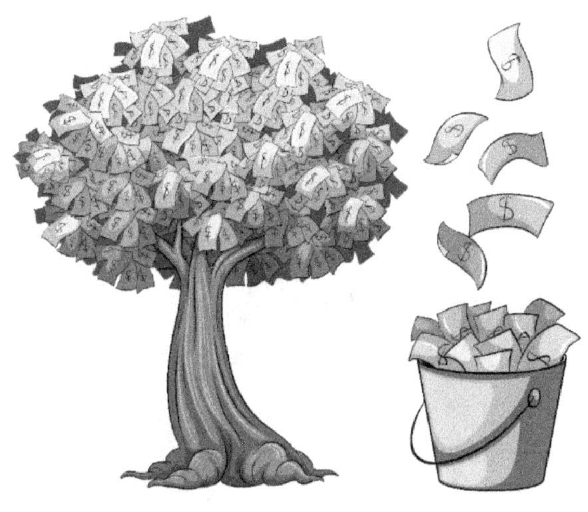

What else can you do if you want to keep living but explore every option to beat this disease? You want to get well and keep living. If emptying your savings is the price you pay for good end results, then so be it. The financial woes of a major illness are stressful at best, but you have to see beyond the dollar marks. It's a hard pill to swallow, but that money in the bank isn't worth a damn if you're not here! Keep your eyes on the prize. Get well and worry about the future IN the future.

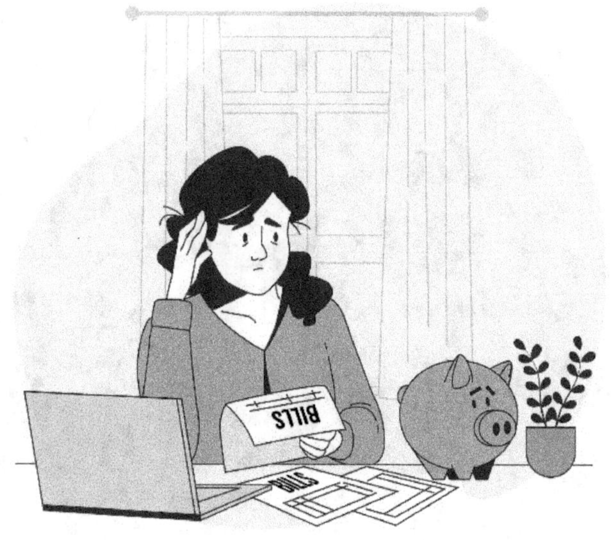

I did some research online to see if there were any groups or foundations available to help breast cancer patients with expenses. Even if your insurance pays well on most things, you may still be responsible for coinsurance and copays. This mounts up and gets out of control quickly. As the statements roll in, it is mind boggling to see in print how much was paid, not to mention how much you still owe.

While talking in the waiting room at the radiation center, many shared stories about searching for financial help with no success. Everyone complains about the astronomical cost of breast cancer treatment and that feeling of 'no end in sight'.

Here are some organizations I found online that are available to assist with financial aid:

The Susan G. Komen Foundation

Pretty In Pink

Patient Advocate Foundation

Please donate when you can so others may get the financial help they so desperately need. Paying medical bills should not be such an enormous burden to someone in the fight for their life, but it's right there in the forefront staring you in the face every day.

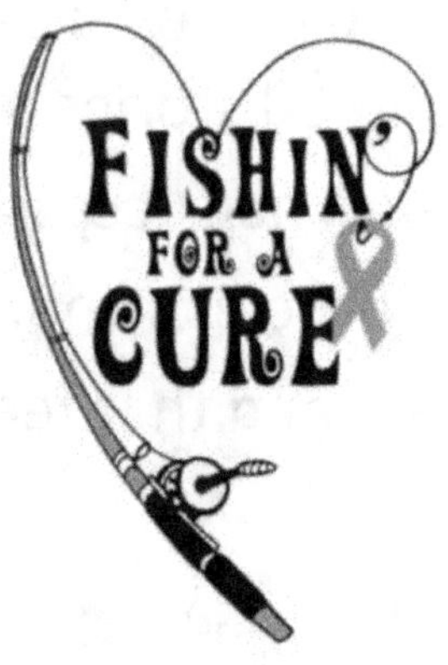

Fishin' For A Cure, Emerald Isle, NC, is a great organization that raises money for breast cancer research through fishing, fun and fellowship. Your donation helps raise awareness of the importance of early detection, as well as fighting to find a cure for women's cancers.

It's great to know organizations like these are working tirelessly to raise money for cancer.

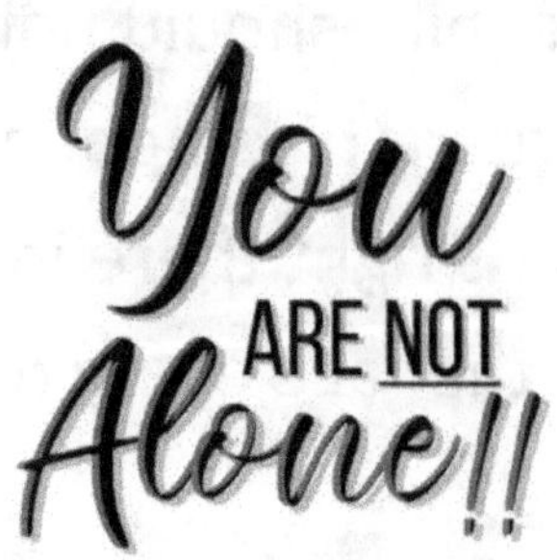

Week 4 of radiation treatments, and I'm burning pretty badly this week. My skin is dark red on my chest and appears almost purple under my arm. It's a little uncomfortable but still tolerable. Heat is radiating from my skin similar to a sunburn. After my recent treatments I go home, take my shirt off, slather up with Aquaphor, and sit there topless to let it cool for a while. The infamous North Carolina heat and humidity in August are not helping my comfort level at all. The temperature outside has been in the 90's for several days. The heat index makes it feels more like 100 to 107 degrees. All these factors together mean one thing: I'm staying inside in the cool!

In the late afternoon when the sun drops behind the trees, most of my backyard is shaded. The cool water in my pool feels so good and soothes my burns for a little while. I'll take that right now. The swim helps to relax me and calms my nerves as well. A change of scenery even for a brief time is welcome.

 The radiation doctor recommended Advil for pain and Aquaphor to be applied topically to the burned areas several times a day. That seems to be working well for now, but I still have 3 more weeks to go. It really feels like a serious sunburn, but I've had those before and suffered through it. I think I can handle this without being a total "wuss."

Week 5 and the burning intensifies every day. I can tolerate it, although it's _really_ painful under my arm and right breast. Sometimes at night it hurts a lot if I roll over the wrong way. I'm hanging in there and suffering through this just knowing it will be over soon. The doctor says I'm doing great and progressing as expected. The farther along I go, the more it feels like wash, rinse, and repeat.

We had new ladies in the waiting room this week to join in with Fannie, Cindy, Paula, and me. Most are coming twice a day for 5 days. Jennie is coming in early this week instead of her normal afternoon appointment. She has a teacher's conference. I guess the variation in radiation treatment depends on what stage of breast cancer you have and the size of your tumor. Each person has a unique treatment plan.

Week 6 and I'm singing ♪♪♪*Burn baby burn, disco inferno!!* ♪♪♪ Woo-wee! It looks and feels like I have a really severe sunburn. At times it becomes very uncomfortable, but I'm hanging in there. Under the arm and under the right breast are the worst areas because its skin touching skin. Aquaphor seems to help a lot, so I'll continue applications and try to stay cool. When it's 82 degrees at 7:00 a.m., you already know it's going to be hotter than hell later in the day. We are under a heat advisory in eastern NC with a heat index of 113. Ugh!! I'll continue to stay inside where it's cool, thank you!

Some days I feel a little nauseated. I have to talk myself out of it, if that makes any sense. I have to be my own coach. I'm determined not to let this get to me, not at all. I get my mind on something else and soon that wave of nausea is gone. I don't have time for all that.

Today is Friday, and I don't have a radiation treatment today. Instead, I get more CT scans. This will be for new mapping and tattoos for my "super boost" of radiation next week. **SUPER BOOST!** I will get the boost all 5 days, and then radiation for me will be done. I feel like I'm in a science fiction movie or possibly a horror movie. It's amazing how this goes on and on and on, but I must persevere to the end. If I'm dreaming, please ...... WAKE UP NOW!!

My completed radiation treatments have focused on the whole breast until now. The upcoming radiation boost will target the area of tissue where the tumor was located, primarily my surgical scar. The goal is to minimize the chances of breast cancer returning. I sure don't want that to happen so bring on the booster. Let's get it done!

My main objective now is to finish radiation and get my post-op mammogram. I pray that it's clear. I want to be through with this forever. That's not too much to ask, is it?
I just want to cross that finish line, a winner, a champion .... a survivor!

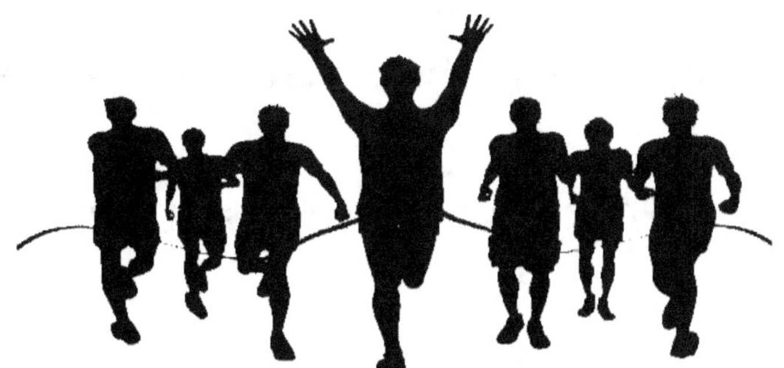

The Finish Line

Drafted into this race, not a volunteer,
It was quite a surprise, to find myself here,
Did my dead-level best to stay with the pace,
Hoping and praying I could win first place.

As I rounded the turns, in record time,
I prayed I would reach the finish line,
With each step I took I strongly believed,
I can win this thing, if I can stay on my feet.

Through tears and pain and determination,
I knew I'd reach my destination,
With patience, faith, and a whole lot of time,
Today with His help, I crossed the finish line!

Written by: Connie Owens August 2023 ©

CHAPTER 7: THE FINISH LINE

Week 7 was finally here, and I was so glad it had arrived. The finish line is near, and I could hardly wait to cross it. Ringing the bell in the lobby of the radiation center is a major milestone for every patient. It signifies their last day of treatment. I'm going to ring that damn bell hard enough to knock it off the wall!! I envisioned it sailing through the lobby, out the windows, through the trees, across the parking lot, and crash landing on someone's windshield! What a glorious day knowing that I have conquered 7 weeks and can put one more part of the journey behind me.

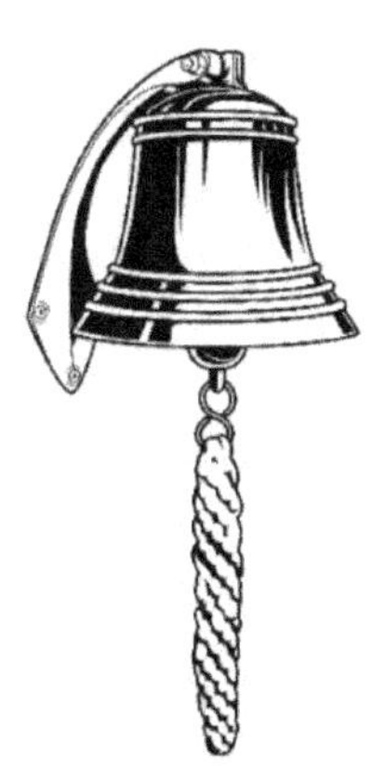

This super boost of radiation continued to burn the already burned skin even more. I prayed the week would go by fast and let the healing of my skin begin quickly. I was ready to heal from all this and get back to some sense of normalcy.

My first day of the boost radiation took more time than usual. Jared and Cindy measured and tweaked and made adjustments to attain exact coordinates before starting the treatment. They explained the importance of precision measurements.

In the middle of week 7, it was time to cue the music and sing along with Johnny Cash...
♪♪♪*And it burns, burns, burns, the ring of fireeeeeee, the ring of fire*♪♪♪! It was quite uncomfortable, but still tolerable if I stayed out of the heat. My saving grace was that it would be over in a few days. The doctor commented that I was progressing well, and my skin looks as

expected and it should start healing in about 2 weeks. The burning of my skin has been in varying shades from purplish black to firetruck red.

Finally the day arrived, my **last** radiation treatment, number **34.** I could SEE the finish line. All the ladies in the waiting room were so nice as they congratulated me on my final day. Fannie, Paula, Cindy, and Ellen still had more days to go, but they will finish soon. It was bittersweet just to know that I wouldn't see all these courageous ladies every morning. Bye, Y'all!

When I was called back to the radiation room, Jared smiled and said, "Don't look to your left." I thought "Hmmmm, wonder why?" When I finished the treatment, I was so surprised to see a bouquet of balloons waiting in the corner. Ashley had brought these in for me this morning as a congratulatory surprise. How sweet was that? Several of the therapists came in to congratulate me and give me a hug. Ashley walked me down to the nurse's station to get my certificate of completion and instructions for care after radiation treatment. They all congratulated me with big smiles. The entire staff here is the greatest! I told them to be on the lookout for my book, I said goodbye to everyone, got dressed and headed to the lobby.

Marsha was waiting in the lobby to take pictures and video my last day. The receptionists, Jackie and Sheena, had big smiles on their faces. People sitting in the lobby stood up to watch what was about to happen. It was exciting!

The moment was here, time to ring the <u>last-day-of-radiation bell</u> and cross the finish line! As a courtesy to everyone working and waiting, I elected not to ring the bell so loud and hard that it fell off the wall, sailed through the lobby, out the windows, through the trees, across the parking lot and crash landed in someone's windshield. In my mind, however, I was swinging on that rope like Quasimodo in *The Hunchback of Notre Dame*! Ha! Everyone in the lobby was smiling and applauding, and I was grinning from ear to ear.

Woo Hoo! Can I get a HELL YEAH? I made it! I survived radiation. I can put that behind me now. I headed home excited and relieved to check off that very last day on my treatment calendar. I earned the luxury to sit back and relax with a big sigh of relief. The final day of radiation is a big accomplishment, and it felt great to say "I did it!" Bring on the marching band!!!

For 34 days I arrived for a 7:45 a.m. treatment. For 34 days I drove a 52-mile round trip. For 34 days I walked 90 steps from the parking lot to the lobby door, and 87 more to the waiting room. For

34 days I laid on the radiation table and listened to 3 ½ songs during treatment. I did this for 7 weeks, 5 days a week, alone. Yes, it became very mundane and repetitious. It felt like the movie *Groundhog Day,* as if every day became the same day on rewind over and over and over for 34 days. Part of me was glad it was over. Another part was going to miss seeing all these wonderful new friends. I hoped all of this was worth it. Time will tell!

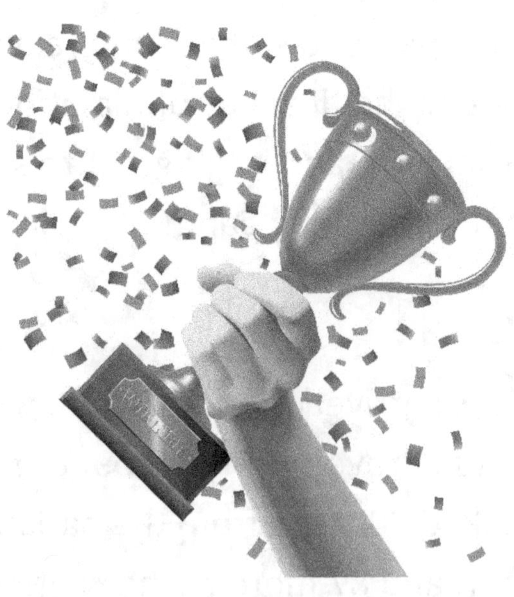

TIME WILL TELL

Radiation is over and I am so glad,
It wasn't fun but it wasn't that bad,
My skin burns, but I'll recover,
I'm not alone, there are many others.

Day by day and week by week,
Even in the hot summer heat,
I sat and waited until my turn,
Knowing each day would increase my burn.

But now at last I say goodbye,
And I'm proud it _never_ made me cry,
My happiest day was ringing the bell,
Was it worth all this?... only Time Will Tell.

Written by: Connie Owens August 2023 ©

CHAPTER 8: TIME WILL TELL

It's been a year now since I was first diagnosed with breast cancer, and what a year it has been. You have followed along with me as I wrote this book chronicling my journey. You know that I went through the mammograms, CT scans, MRIs, bone scans, X-rays, blood work, chemo, biopsy prescriptions drugs, surgery, and radiation. I had pain, depression, lack of energy, hair thinning, was lonely as hell, burned like hell, and just didn't feel like going anywhere or doing anything. Even with all that behind me, I'm still not completely out of the woods. I had to see what my oncologist recommended for the next steps in preventive care. I guess time will tell if all this treatment has worked.

One thing I know is, you must psych your mind from the onset at diagnosis, and continually reinforce your mindset toward survival. You have to be bold, courageous, and firm in your own convictions that you will prevail as <u>victorious</u> at the journey's end. You must persevere with that determination every hour of every day. I know I have. I told myself early on, "Girl, you are strong enough to beat this thing." Through all the appointments, doctors, prescriptions, surgery, radiation, and all the tests, I told myself, _"Connie you can and you will stand strong!"_ **Miss Connie has spoken!**

You must strive to always have positive vibes for yourself and around others. Don't let family and friends dread talking to you because you sound so depressed and negative all the time. I tried to remain as upbeat and positive as I could through all of this.

When asked how I felt, I was truthful, but I never delved into all the fine details of how I really felt. There is nothing anyone can do so why burden them with all that. Suck it up and shut up!

My best friend, Jackie, told me this, and I totally agree: *"Remember this, a "woe-as-me" pity party does not help you or anyone else so don't go there. It's easy to fall into that pattern, but it's not good for you. Depressing as all of this is, dragging that albatross around is an added burden to everyone."*

I knew a follow-up mammogram was to follow shortly after radiation was completed, and I couldn't wait to see if the results were good. This would be the first mammogram since surgery and radiation.

I couldn't wait to feel a rush of relief and exhilaration if it was good news. I felt I had earned that feeling. After all, this had been one hell of a long roller-coaster ride that I couldn't get off and hope to never ride again. I couldn't begin to grasp the mere sense of defeat and dread that I would feel if something looked "suspicious."

I'm a tough ole gal, but my God, my resilience had been tested through and through. It's amazing the strength you can find from within to fight the fight of your life. I never really knew before what a cancer patient endures, although I now understand why they call sick people "patients." You must have the "patience of **Job**" and a bottomless pit of tenacity to go through all these phases of various treatments in order to get well. I have been a "patient patient." (not)

The English language is so strange. It's funny that two words spelled alike can have totally different meanings when used as either an adjective or a noun. As an **adjective** "patient" means; *able to accept or tolerate delays, problems, or suffering without becoming annoyed or anxious*. As a **noun** "patient" means; *a person receiving or registered to receive medical treatment.* Hmm that's deep. Ok, so I drifted off there for a moment, sorry.

Finally the day arrived, the day I would get my tell-tale mammogram. I must admit my anxiety level was about to go into overdrive. Of all things, a hurricane came on shore in Florida this week, turned into a tropical storm, and was now wreaking havoc on North Carolina. Gusty winds, pouring rain, alerts going off on my cell phone warning of flash flooding, and I wondered what else could happen. Really? I mean REALLY?? The hits just keep coming. Since my tornado drama, everyone who knows me knows how I feel when a storm develops and understands how my nerves are affected.

I had endured a lot in this past year. Through all the ups and downs of receiving an unexpected medical diagnosis that shocked me to my core and the subsequent treatments involved with it, I would not be deterred from making this appointment today. The moment of truth was near, and there was nothing that would keep me from getting to the clinic and having this mammogram today. Say it with me, "<u>NOTHING</u>!"

In a couple of hours, I would have it all done and get the results, but most importantly I would see the images. They say a picture is worth a thousand words. I think if all looks good, I'm confident that I will find more than a thousand words to describe my feelings about it. Everyone who knows me knows I like to talk (a lot). I'm pretty sure I won't stop talking about this for quite some time.

The drive over wasn't too bad. It was raining with some wind gusts but nothing out of the ordinary. I arrived, checked in, and waited to be call back. A man was filling out a crossword puzzle while he waited for someone, and he kept clicking his ball point pen. It was quite annoying to me, and I noticed others cutting their eyes over at him thinking exactly what I was thinking.

 Finally, another nearby lady spoke up and said, "Sir, I hate to ask you this, but would you not click that pen?" He apologized immediately and said he wasn't aware he was doing it. He also added that the same thing would get on his nerves. Several in the waiting room laughed and snickered. I was thinking, 'thank you'. <u>Today</u> was not the day to be tested. I didn't need to be charged with assault before I had this very important mammogram. Ha!

After a short wait I was called back, I put on a gown, and then proceeded into the room for a diagnostic mammogram. The technician explained that today I would get a different type mammogram than usual because of my lumpectomy. This machine would be taking 3-D images and magnified images to be sure nothing was hiding in there. I was informed that I would get a mammogram like this for the next 3 years.

It was over quickly, and I asked if I could see the images. She showed me each image, and I asked if there was anything I should be concerned about. She said, "No, everything looks great." Hallelujah! Finally, I can see the results of this very long, painful year. I left there slightly in shock but very happy. I needed to sit in my car a few minutes and collect my thoughts.

Peggy had warned me, out of nowhere at some point in time, that I was going to have a good cry. She went through this a few years ago, and she said it will release all that tension built up in you. She assured me that it would eventually happen!

Well today was the day. I sat in my car in that parking lot and had a good ole' thank-you-Jesus cry. After taking a few more minutes to compose myself, a lunch treat at Chick-fil-A seemed in order to top off the day before heading home!

Another week passed before I had a follow-up appointment with the surgeon to discuss the mammogram results. He reported that the mammogram was clean, no signs of anything abnormal. He did an exam and said all was good, He suggested that I continue to do self-breast exams regularly.

Next, I saw my oncologist, and she was most excited that the mammogram was clear and showed no cancer or benign tumors. As a continuing precaution, she now wants to prescribe Letrozole once a day and Verzenio twice a day.

Letrozole is a hormone blocker and Verzenio helps kill cancer cells that may have been left behind after surgery, chemotherapy, and radiation to help prevent recurrence. Both will have some side effects. I'm dreading taking the pills, but if this is what I must do to stay cancer free, I'll do it. This was an exciting day to have both doctors say to me, "no signs of cancer!" <u>CANCER FREE</u>! Finally!!

We all know that everyone has a busy schedule with work and family, but please remember that a cancer patient feels all alone and feels that the rest of the world is going on without them. We are scared, and our whole existence has been upended. It's the smallest of things that make the biggest difference in a day that is just not going well.

While talking with the women in the waiting room, someone asked, "What have you learned from all of this?" It was somewhat surprising that **everyone** said the same thing, <u>"I found out who I can depend on."</u> You really do find out, and it's an eye opener. It's also very sad.

After all I have experienced, I can hopefully offer some words of wisdom and a birds-eye view perspective concerning cancer patients and their emotional state. Please remember the following things if you have a family member or if you know someone who has cancer. Be the hero!

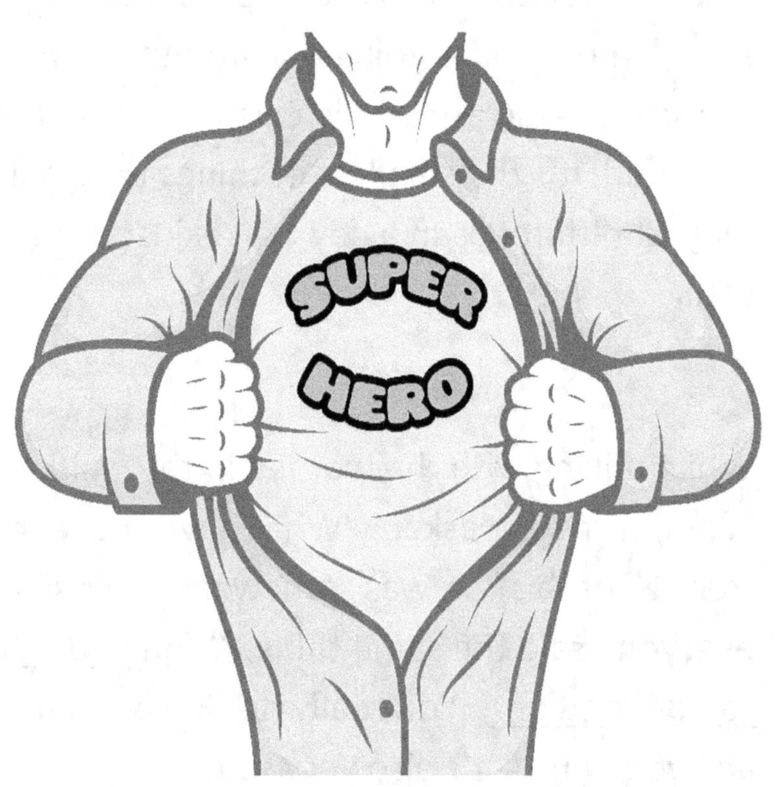

.

C - **<u>Check</u>** on them frequently. Email, text, or <u>c</u>all. It will make a difference knowing you <u>c</u>are. They will remember this <u>always</u>.

A - **<u>Ask</u>** them, "What can I do for you?" or, "I'm going to town, do you need anything?" Be supportive and show you have their back. Don't say, "I'll be there for you" and then *not be there*.

N – **<u>Never</u>**, <u>n</u>ever say, "Well it could have been worse!" Theres no doubt it could have been, but those are <u>n</u>ot words of encouragement, <u>n</u>ot at all. It's better to say <u>n</u>othing than to say that.

C – **<u>Cook</u>** a meal or stop for <u>c</u>arry-out and take it to them. That is a sure way to make them smile and feel better. There's nothing like <u>c</u>omfort food, especially from a friend or family member.

E – **<u>Excite</u>** them with a small trinket or gift, just something to show you are thinking of them. Something they can look at, treasure, and know that your care is priceless.

R – **<u>Remember</u>** their appointment dates. Call, and say, "Good luck tomorrow!" Ask how treatment went today. It makes them feel good that you are keeping up with their schedule.

I went on a 14-day trip to Greece in the spring of 2022. I had a great time, and I met a lot of wonderful new friends along the way. Little did I know 3 months after I returned that my life would be turned upside down, and I wouldn't be able to go anywhere like that for quite a while. Hopefully one day soon I can. Time will tell.

I saw some beautiful sites and visited a lot of historical places. I stood at the original Olympic stadium in Olympia, and I even climbed those steep stairs in Athens to get to the top of the Acropolis and see the Parthenon. I was overcome with the beauty and awe of all these things. I'm so glad I have all that imprinted in my mind forever. They are wonderful memories to reflect on. The new friends I met on this trip have stayed in touch with me throughout this journey.

Knowing that life can change in the blink of an eye and there's nothing you can do to stop it, makes you see everything in a new way. In other words, be sure to stop and smell the roses. I know I will from this day forward.

Thank you to everyone who prayed for me, called on the phone, texted me, sent cards, provided meals, and sent gifts. Also, to those who came by to visit, checked on me, and did my yardwork when I just couldn't, thank you. Thank you all so very much!

Thank you to my family and closest friends for moral support. Thank you, Jackie, for the hours and hours of edits.

Thank you so much to all the doctors and their staffs. The professional care I received throughout this journey has been wonderful. You prescribed the best treatments for my chance to beat this horrible disease.

CONCLUSION

Breast cancer is the second cause of cancer related deaths in the U. S., second only to lung cancer. Statistics show that breast cancer is typically diagnosed in older women, with the median age being around 63, but it is also diagnosed in younger women. I was **70** when mine was diagnosed. PLEASE go get your annual mammograms no matter your age. I know, we all hate it, sure we do, but it can save you a lot of time and money in the long run.

<u>Early detection can SAVE YOUR LIFE!</u>

THE END

Connie Owens

Please feel free to email me at:
ritesongs@gmail.com

"You gain strength, courage, and confidence by every experience in which you really stop to look fear in the face. You are able to say to yourself, 'I have lived through this horror. I can take the next thing that comes along.' You must do the thing you think you cannot do."

— **Eleanor Roosevelt, (1960)** <u>**You Learn by Living: Eleven Keys for a More Fulfilling Life**</u>

All illustrations designed by Freepik.com

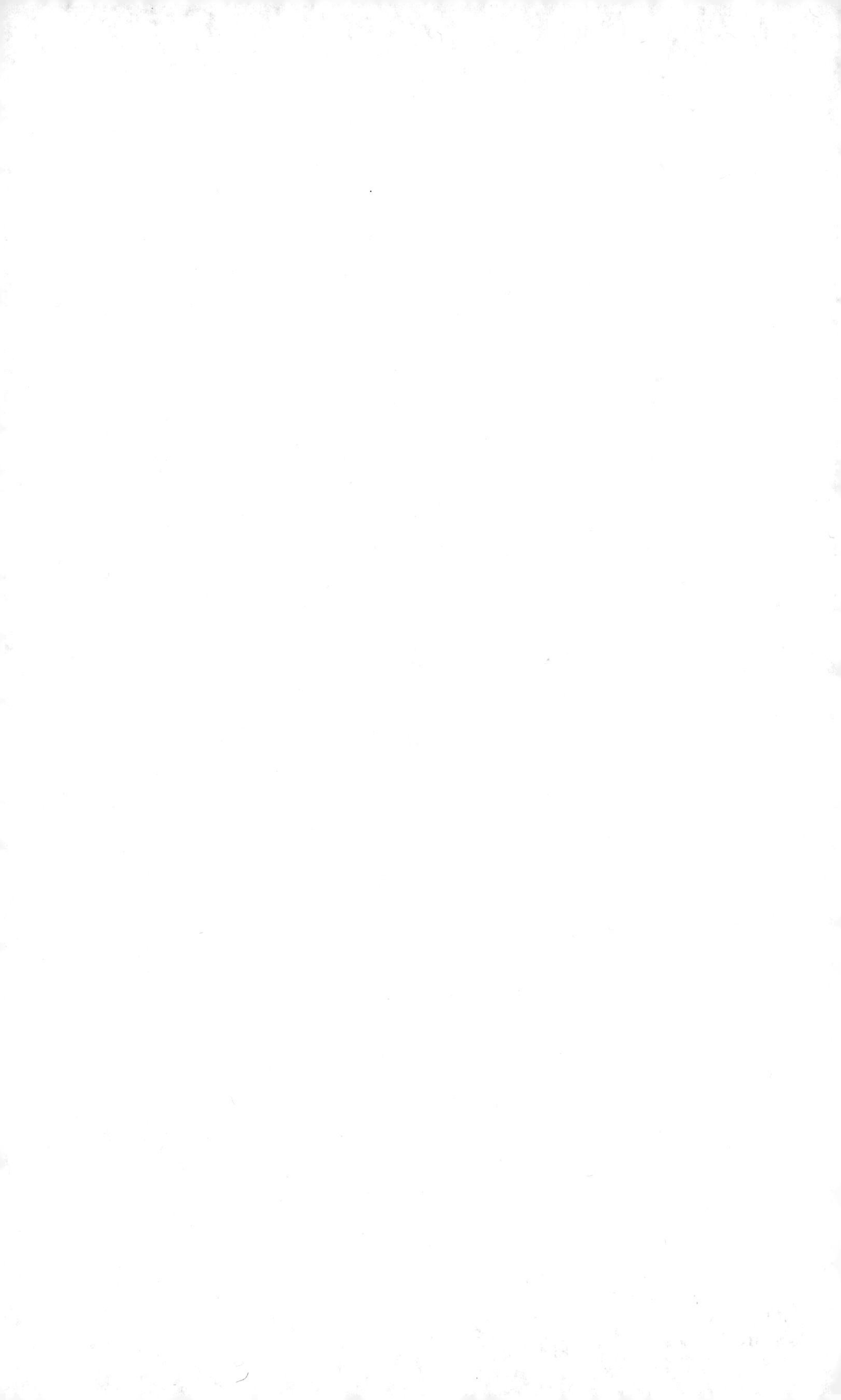